Contents

CW00428138

Forward

I wrote this booklet in 2007 but it was way back in the early 1990's that I eventually discovered that three natural ingredients could help me with my irritable bowel syndrome.

It became very clear to me that the three ingredients that I refer to in the booklet - namely psyllium husks, inulin and a blend of probiotic cultures - worked better when taken together than individually.

In other words they all had a synergy with each other.

There was no research to back this theory up at the time – none existed. The breakthrough of finding that the three ingredients could really work took me three years to work out.

In the section on prebiotics, I have already mentioned how research in the last few years has proven that inulin can enhance and protect the activity of probiotics in the colon.

This is now known in scientific circles as the 'symbiotic' effect.

This is significant because often the secret to finding success in overcoming bowel disease is restoring a good bacterial balance.

Sounds simple enough but it isn't. I know that many people take copious amount of probiotics without any noticeable improvements to bowel health.

If the environment within your bowels is unstable and there is no consistency to bowel movements and formation, then probiotics can struggle to get a foothold and do their job.

This is where psyllium husks come into their own.

I am now delighted to say that in the last two years, two separate studies have proven the important role that psyllium husks can play in overcoming irritable bowel syndrome and ulcerative colitis.

Both inulin and psyllium husks can help to support the restoration of probiotics in different ways and studies – at long last - are now showing that this trinity of ingredients can really make a difference when taken together.

The role of psyllium husks

The two recent studies have demonstrated the important role psyllium husks can play in irritable bowel syndrome.

One of the most significant studies was carried out in Japan. This study showed that when probiotics were taken by ulcerative colitis sufferers, very few benefits were shown but when probiotics were taken with psyllium husks, the quality of life of the sufferers was markedly improved.

This was a randomised controlled trial carried out at the Nippon Medical School Tokyo on the efficacy of symbiotic versus probiotic or prebiotic treatment to improve the quality of life in patients with ulceratvie colitis.' Authors: S. Fujimori, K. Gudis, K. Mitsui, T. Seo, M. Yonezawa, S.Tanaka, A. Tatguchi, C. Sakamoto. doi:10.1016/j.nut.2008.11.017

This study proved my theory way back in 1994 that taking probiotics and psyllium worked when taken together but had little effect when taken individually.

It's nice to see my original theories now proven by real research!

It has always been my belief that psyllium husks are capable of providing the ability that the probiotics need to 'regroup.' No other fibre – in my experience – has the capability to do this in such an efficient way.

As I mention throughout the booklet, when psyllium is added to water, it forms a soft gel which is suitable for even the most sensitive of systems.

As this gel makes its way through the digestive tract, it maintains a moist environment which is just what the healthy bacteria need to thrive in.

It is my belief that the gel becomes a 'protected' environment for the bacteria – a sort of shield. The inulin gives further support by acting as a readily available source of food for the good bacteria to proliferate.

Dutch study

Another recent study – this time in Holland - has further pinpointed the role of psyllium husks in improving bowel health. The Dutch study compared the use o psyllium husks against bran fibre in cases of irritable bowel syndrome.

They found that psyllium husks had significant benefits for sufferers whereas bra fibre, in most cases, made things worse.

As I have always said, psyllium husks have a very gentle 'chamois leather' effec on cleansing the bowels whereas bran fibre works more like an abrasive brillo pa

To quote the main researcher in the Dutch study, Dr Niek de Wit:

'It is unlikely that people with IBS would get enough soluble fibre from fruit and other foods to help them. I thing adding psyllium to the diet is the best treatmen option to start with. In the study, people did this by adding it to things such as yoghurt and it had real effect.'

Bijkerk CJ et al, Soluble or insoluble fibre in irritable bowel syndrome in prima care. Randomised placebo controlled trial. BMJ 2009;339 (Aug 27)

Whatever your level of knowledge of food and nutrition, I hope you've found thi report to be enlightening and helpful. Please let me know about your experience dealing with IBS, and any suggestions you may have for improving the report content.

Kind regards

Peter Jackson

Introduction

irst of all, I would like to introduce myself. My name is Peter Jackson and I have een involved commercially in the alternative health business for many years.

fter a very long period of stress, backed up with extensive travel in far away laces, I found myself with a condition that I now know to be sensitive Irritable owel Syndrome. I say sensitive, because it was the 'loose' variety for most of ie time where I was rushing to the loo a few times a day, although this was interspersed with constipation.

was given various bits of advice on how to tackle my predicament, and one of em was to increase my fibre. At that time, fibre to me meant more wheat fibre so went out and purchased wheat bran to put on my cereals and into my soup.

ie direct consequence of this was that my symptoms got much worse even though e original cause of my stress was no longer an issue. Nothing seemed to give any al relief. I was starting to lose weight and was feeling tired most of the time. It as clear that I was not digesting my food or absorbing nutrients effectively.

rtunately for me, I had some background in the health trade and I decided to see if ere was anything that I might do with my diet to help. I spent some time reviewing e latest research on diet and nutrients and in the end found a combination of things at really worked for me.

iings have moved on since then, but the original combination of foods and gredients that helped me back then are still doing so today.

ie main idea of this book is to pass on my experiences and also to give you some ʻormation on your diet and other nutrients that may be useful to long term bowel alth.

vas absolutely clear to me that, without good bowel health, my whole body couldn't iction. Indeed most of the practitioners I consulted at the time were adamant that if u want to enjoy robust, good health, this can only be achieved if the Colon, the part the digestive system that expels waste, is, itself, clean and healthy.

If the Colon is not healthy, then toxins can build up within the body which, if n
checked, can affect overall health. 'Leaky Gut' is a term which is starting to
more widely used.

Certainly my health was suffering. On my quest to learn more, I was soon to lea
that poor digestion and elimination is to blame for a host of modern ailments, y
most of these are preventable. It is generally felt that 80% of bowel cancers a
preventable and so it is fairly safe to assume that diet and lifestyle does play a maj
part in bowel disease.

During my quest to learn more about the health of the bowels, I came across th
quote from a well known nutritionist:

*'Most middle aged people have between three and fifteen pounds of undigest
faecal matter stuck in their colon. Waste matter which gets stuck in the Colon
highly toxic and suppresses the immune system, potentially causing gas, bloati
and a sluggish digestive system dramatically reducing the assimilation of nutrier
and slowing metabolism.'*

Our digestive system is the focal point of our bodies, and the ability to abso
nutrients from our food is the key to our survival. What is more, a healthy digesti
system is vital for our general well-being, and many illnesses and allergies can
traced to underlying intestinal problems.

Many experts believe impacted waste material in the bowel can harden and
thicken over the years restricting the colon passage and limiting the amount of
nutrients that can be absorbed from the foods we eat.

Constipation is a western problem. And now, so are IBS, Diverticulitis, laxative
addiction, anal fissures, haemorrhoids, sluggishness, fatigue, bloating and so on.
Is this just a coincidence?

Education, understanding and implementing what we learn will help us resolve th
digestive issues we are dealing with on a daily basis.

When I first started to talk about my problem, bowels were very much a 'taboo' subje

Happily, more than 10 years on, things are much more out in the open.

the UK, the government has declared one week each year as 'gut week' in a bid
raise awareness of the importance of gut health and to encourage prevention and
rly diagnosis of problems.

s clear that keeping your bowels healthy is far easier said than done for most of
with the stressful and busy lives we lead. In my case stress, along with long
riods of travel in 3rd world countries where the food was sometimes a bit 'iffy' I
scovered that it was not always possible to eat a great diet.

id discover however that there were certain natural ingredients that I could take
my travels that did have a direct, positive affect on how my bowels behaved.

oon realised that achieving normal bowel transit time was vital to my bowel and
imately overall health.

wever, before going into detail about these ingredients, it is important to look
your diet to see how the food you eat could have a direct effect on your bowel
alth.

How healthy is your diet?

If your diet is perfect there is a good chance that your health will be as we
Our bowels are likely to be directly affected by our diet over time.

Just by eating lots of fresh vegetables you can improve your bowel health becau
vegetables, in particular leeks, garlic, onions and artichokes, have a 'prebiot
effect in your bowels. This means they help you produce your own good bacter
which is very important to bowel health.

You can learn more about this later on when I talk about healthy bacteria.

In recent years, many more of us are now understanding that food is our medici
and what we eat can have a profound effect on our health. However, if your life
fast, you may rely on a prepared meal for most of your daily food requirements, a
this often means consuming 'dead' food which has little in the way of antioxida
activity and virtually no fibre.

It is no coincidence that some hospitals have constipation clinics for children under 6!!!

This would not have been heard of even 30 years ago, but have you analysed son
of the fast food children eat? It is loaded with fat and has no fibre whatsoever. Fib
is vital for bowel health and you can see more about this in the fibre section. If yo
eat a perfect diet, then you will consume lots of fibre.

The fact that most of us don't get near the recommended levels of 26 - 35g of fibre p
day says that most of us for one reason or another are not eating enough fresh food

So, your overall diet is crucial, but there is a well known statement which says th
it's not what you eat, it's what you absorb!

So, lets look at your digestion first.

Chew your food
Our digestive systems are amazing things. They process the food we eat and exp
the waste at the other end. But sometimes, factors such as stress, ill health, gettin
older or today's process diets may mean that an optimum digestive system isn
something everyone enjoys every day.

f you add to this the fact that millions of people in the UK shovel highly processed od into their mouths without even bothering to chew it properly, then it is not urprising that the biggest section in pharmacy is often devoted to products for adigestion.

Often, the typical OTC product just masks the symptoms rather than looks at the ause of the problem in the first place.

is not the purpose of this book to give you details of every step of the digestion rocess but it is certainly worth mentioning the one part of the digestive process that ou can have direct control over – chewing.

hewing is the first part of the digestive process and people don't do enough of it. ood lubrication is needed to combine digestive enzymes with food and to help osorption of nutrients. Saliva lubricates food, making it easier to swallow. It is so rich in a digestive enzyme that breaks down carbohydrates.

urther on in the digestive process, other enzymes are secreted by the pancreas and ver to aid the digestion through the gut, but the whole process will work better if ou 'liquidise' your foods in the mouth first.

hilst on the subject of chewing, it is worth talking about when to drink round a eal. The ideal scenario is probably to be well hydrated before a meal. This means inking around 25-30 minutes before eating. In this way you should not be thirsty ring a meal.

rinking too much during a meal can dilute the digestive enzymes and therefore pede good digestion. Of course, as with all things, there is a balance to be made re. I'm not saying don't drink anything at all and of course don't stop drinking e wine in moderation, but if you can keep drinking during your meal down to a inimum, then this would be the best plan of action.

rinking coffee or tea immediately after a meal is also not the best policy for the me reason. Giving yourself a break of around 30 minutes before taking a drink ould be the best option.

any don't realise that a healthy digestive system and healthy bowels are closely nnected. When food is broken down more efficiently it makes it easier to digest d this means that not only are vital nutrients better absorbed in the small intestine, t waste matter is also passed through more easily by the bowels.

Food which remains undigested, may in fact become an irritant to the large bowel So chew your soup and drink your solids! -   this is good advice – make sure tha your food is as liquid as possible before swallowing!

To summarise:

1. Chew your food slowly and thoroughly and make it as liquid as possible. This reduces the stress on the digestive system and encourages the secretion of the all important digestive enzymes.
2. Eating too quickly can cause excess gas, so keep your mouth closed whil chewing! (Others will appreciate it). Bloatedness in the abdomen can be a sign of trapped gas.
3. Don't eat too late at night.
4. Rest after each meal
5. Eat small meals, and reduce fat in the meal as much as possible.

'The early bird may get the worm, but the second mouse gets the cheese. This o Zen saying should apply to how you eat your food – Don't rush it!

Digestive enzyme supplementation can be useful at certain times when the digestiv process is under stress.

The Food You Eat

So, chewing your food well and taking your time over eating is the first step to tak The next is trying to eat a well rounded diet. I don't like to use the work 'balance because it is so over used. The reality is that for one reason or another, very few o us seem to get it right.

I was preparing to list all the 'do's and don'ts' of a diet for bowel health but then ju last week I learned of a new study from France which really did the job for me.

The study confirmed earlier findings that the high calorie, low fibre foods associate with the Western diet are associated with an increased risk of colon cancer.
This is not the first time that such dietary habits have been linked to increased ri of bowel cancer. According to the British charity Cancer Research UK:

"Countries that have had a rapid 'westernisation' of diet, such as Japan, have see a rapid increase in the incidence of colorectal cancer. Consumption of meat an dairy products in Japan increased ten-fold between the 1950s and 1990s."

e new research, published in the *American Journal of Epidemiology*, was based
the French cohort of the European Prospective Investigation into Cancer and
itrition (EPIC) study.

o explain this: Throughout Europe, there are long term studies underway to
termine the effects that different diets have on peoples' health. I believe I am
rrect in saying that this massive project is being managed from the UK. Different
dies, taking place over many years, are being carried out across many countries.
is particular study was carried out in France and relates to diets and their influence
bowel health).

ur dietary patterns were identified by the author of the study.

A diet rich in fruit and vegetables, lots of olive oil, and fish. This is fairly
nilar to a 'Mediterranean diet.' This is the diet which is considered to be the most
althy for the bowels. In fact the consumption of fish has been shown to have
rticular benefits for bowel health. Also, if you are vegetarian, you are far less
ely to get bowel cancer than red meat eaters.

A Western diet. This is a diet rich in processed meat, eggs, butter, potatoes,
ocessed grain products, and cheese. This diet was associated with a 39 % increase
bowel disease.

The 'drinker' diet. Here there is an emphasis on alcoholic consumption, snacks,
ndwiches and processed meat. This diet was associated with a 42% increase in
wel disease.

'Meat eaters'' (meat and poultry). Here the risk rose to 58%. Here the emphasis
on red meat.

e conclusions of this summary are therefore fairly clear.

heat
general, the best advice appears to be to keep wheat intake low. The intake of gluten
wheat over many years is reckoned to be one of the causes of bowel problems. Our
gestive systems are not used or designed to eat processed white bread.

hite bread is made from fine roller milled flour that is produced so quickly that
starch it contains remains wrapped up and so our digestive enzymes are unable
get into it. Consequently we end up with undigested food passing into the colon
d lower bowel.

Bread made from traditional stone ground flour is easier to digest because t
millstones crack open the wheat, allowing our digestive enzymes to reach t
starch. This can be particularly important for old people who may not be producii
digestive enzymes so effectively.

Caffeine
Caffeine should also be kept to a minimum as it is an irritant and messes up yo
energy cycle.

Water
Don't forget the water, drink an extra 2 litres per day, it's good for your bowels
well as general health.

Exercise
And finally, bad news for those of you who don't like exercise. Research in Taiw;
at the Chang Gung University has concluded that exercise also significantly reduc
colon cancer. No real reason is known for this but an assumption can be ma
that athletes defecate more than none athletes (exercise tends to enhance intestin
motility).

This more frequent defecation pattern decreases the period of time that potenti
carcinogens in the colon are actually in contact with the lining of the colon.

It's all about balance…….

In this section I have just given a few pointers on some 'do's and 'don'ts.' As yo
can see, a diet that is good for the bowels is going to be good for your heart as we
so there is good reason to aim towards the Mediterranean type of diet.

No one is going to get it 100% right, it just means getting the balance in yo
favour. This probably means that around 80% of your diet should be made up
things that are recognised as being good for your bowels, keeping the 20% for son
indulgence!

One thing you can't ignore in your diet is fibre. Most of us don't get enough, a;
there is one fibre that I have found to be absolutely brilliant in keeping my digesti
system regular and in good condition…..

Soluble fibre and its emergence as *the* fibre

Apparently there are five different types of fibre, but you will find there are two you will hear about most, they are soluble and insoluble fibre.

In short, bran fibre like wheat bran is classified as insoluble fibre. It is not water retentive but can stimulate bowels by a natural process of 'scratching' the bowel wall as it moves through, therefore stimulating a peristalsis movement.

Whereas this process is perfectly natural, you can imagine that this 'scratching' effect could make a sensitive situation worse, as I found out to my cost.

Soluble fibre by contrast has more absorbent qualities and tends to be more water retentive and therefore more viscous. This viscous quality makes it more 'gentle' on the digestive system and, in most cases, is better for people with sensitive bowels than insoluble fibre. A typical example of soluble fibre is oats.

But Fibre is not only about relieving constipation. I needed a fibre supplement to help me overcome my prolonged period of diarrhoea. Getting fibre from your diet is of course the best option for anyone. But there may be times in your life when fibre supplementation might be necessary and this is when you need to know what is the best fibre for you.

Over the last 100 years our demands for and interest in fibre have gone through some changes. Below I have given a very brief summary of what has been going on.

A brief history of fibre in the 20th Century!!

Our grandparents and their parents enjoyed far higher levels of fibre in their diet because they ate a lot more fresh food with higher levels of naturally occurring fibre. The advantage of getting fibre in this way is that high fibre foods like whole grains contain not only lots of fibre but also other beneficial nutrients and antioxidants.

Also, our great grandparents were far more likely to have consumed whole wheat bread. Having lots of fibre means lower transit time and this, it seems, means less bowel disease.

Once white bread became fashionable in the 1930's and 40's, fibre almost became a forgotten word. White bread was even considered by many to be better for you than whole wheat. People however were still getting reasonable amounts of fibre from their general diet.

It wasn't until the 1970's that fibre started to make a comeback. It was then that a Dr Birkett from the UK started to study the diet of black Africans who had virtually no bowel disease, compared to western Europe where the disease was increasing.

To cut a long story short, Dr Birkett discovered the main difference between the two diets was the level of fibre. Needless to say, the levels of fibre in the black African diet was far higher than the western diet. The fibre came mainly from whole grains which also had the benefits of extra nutrients and antioxidants.

After this study, and his book was published, people started to eat more fibre. And you could buy big bags of wheat bran fibre in health shops to add to your cereal.

This continued into the 1980's when the demand for fibre exploded with publication of The F Plan Diet. It was at the time that fibre supplements started but most of these tended to be based on wheat and insoluble fibre.

Then the 90's came with more written about low fat and low calorie diets and fibre once again took a back seat.

However, since 2000, fibre has made a big comeback in the USA and this has started to filter through over here in the UK. This time the news is not so much about insoluble fibre, it's all to do with soluble fibre.

In the US, the general recommendation is that everyone should consume 35 g of fibre per day and the emphasis is definitely on soluble fibre. It is stated that most people consume less than half of this. (Not surprising when you look at their fast food diet). The US authorities are trying to get people to consume more soluble fibre as it is generally considered that this type of fibre reduces the risk of obesity, type 2 diabetes and also colon cancer.

In the case of Type 2 Diabetes, soluble fibre, because of its absorbent qualities, may control blood sugar by delaying gastric emptying, retarding the entry of glucose into the blood stream and lessening the post meal rise in blood sugar.

The cholesterol lowering effect of soluble fibres may also help those with diabetes by reducing heart disease risks. It appears that soluble fibre reduces cholesterol because of the gel it forms once mixed with water.

As it passes through the digestive tract, the gel traps some substances related to high cholesterol. There is some evidence that this process may lessen heart disease risks because of the reduced amount of cholesterol that is absorbed into the blood stream.

Studies find that people on high fibre diets have lower total cholesterol levels and may be less likely to form harmful blood clots than those who consume low fibre diets. A recent USA report found that, in sufficient amounts, fibre apparently reduced heart disease risks among men who ate more than 25 grams per day, compared to those consuming under 15 grams per day.

Fibre and weight loss

Recent research from Tufts University in the US suggests that people trying to lose weight should also consider placing greater emphasis on something as simple as fibre in their diet.

In the research it was found that in the case of women in particular, those with low levels of fibre in their diet were far more likely to be overweight. Obesity was measured by the BMI (body mass index).

It was found that there was a direct correlation between fibre intake and BMI, the higher the levels of fibre, the lower the BMI. Also, having more fibre in your diet lowers the glycaemic index of food, as it helps to slow the release of carbohydrates into the blood stream. I touched on this earlier.

My quest for the right type of fibre.

Whilst I was struggling with my bowels, I wanted to try and find a natural way to slow things down.' I was starting to improve my diet, but this was not having a dramatic effect on things.

I was advised to look at soluble fibre as the most natural way of slowing things. In the 90's not so much was known about soluble fibre so I needed to experiment myself. I tried guar gum, konjac fibre, oat beta glucan (extracts from oats) and whilst these were helpful in slowing things down marginally, I still was not getting the results I required.

I then tried Isphagula husk from the doctor which was an improvement over the other fibres and I felt as though I was getting there but even here there was little bulk to my stools.

. At last I found what I was looking for when I was recommended whole psyllium husks by a Dutch Naturopath. This fibre is related to isphagula husk. The whole psyllium husks were in their natural husk form which meant that they were not ground down to a fine powder.

I found the whole husks far more tolerable for a sensitive system like mine.

In my view, whole psyllium husk is the 'Rolls Royce' of all fibres. It definitely helped me to get more bulk to my stools and slowed down my transit time in a totally natural way.

The great thing is that this fibre is also fantastic for constipation as well.

Although this would appear illogical, whole psyllium husk can also help in a 'sluggish' situation as well where waste matter may have been hanging around too long.

The extra bulk the fibre offers gives the bowel wall something to work on, thus encouraging the Peristalsis action. When added to water, Psyllium absorbs 25 times its own weight in water. The gel that is formed acts like a very gentle broom and this helps to keep the bowels clear.

This can be important because dry, hard stools over a prolonged period can be one of the causes of many bowel problems.

A 'moist' stool is far easier and more comfortable to pass.

This is why my preferred fibre is the soluble type. If stools are easier to pass, this means there is less straining and far less likelihood of haemorrhoids and Diverticular disease (when small pouches, sacs or pocket-like openings develop in the colon or bowel walls).

Also, this moist environment that is created, promotes the type of fertile conditions in which healthy bacteria can flourish, helping to prevent dysbiosis, a situation where bad bacteria gets the upper hand.

More Water
As we are made of water, we depend on it as a transport system within our bodies. A person can exist several weeks without solid food, but will die within a few days without water. We need to drink eight to ten glasses of the best quality water available per day in order to maintain health.

I wanted to talk about water here because if you do decide to increase your fibre-in-take it is very important to increase your water as well.

Water is a good way to detoxify your system. It is now recognised that we do not drink sufficient, preferring instead to drink coffee and tea, both of which are diuretics which can lead to dehydration.

Taking extra water is particularly important if you are taking extra fibre in your diet. Fibre absorbs water to give more bulk and this is important to improve the peristaltic action of the bowels. (Fibre without enough water can = cement. So, don't forget the water)!

So, get as much fibre as you can from your diet – but if you need to supplement for whatever reason or you want to increase fibre to make sure you get your 35g fibre per day, the fibre I recommend is Psyllium.

But good bowel health may need more than just the right type of fibre, it also needs lots of friendly bacteria (Probiotic Cultures)....

Friendly Bacteria – make sure your system gets plenty of variety

You will of course have heard lots about how important friendly bacteria is to our bowels, our immune system and long term health.

Put simply, having lots of friendly bacteria in your guts reduces the chance of any bad bacteria getting a hold and it is this process that reduces the risk of bowel problems. More friendly bacteria means a bowel that is more resistant to infection.

This is why it is good advice to take a probiotic supplement a few weeks before you go on holiday. It will reduce your chance of tummy upsets.

Many nutritionists now believe that long term deficiency of good bacteria is considered to be the start of bowel disease. Certainly long term use of antibiotics, because they kill good as well as bad bacteria, is now considered to be one of the potential causes of deficiencies of friendly bacteria.

If you are taking antibiotics therefore, try and take probiotics as well. The secret is to take the probiotics at a different time to when you take the antibiotics. A couple of hours should be sufficient to make sure the antibiotics don't wipe out the probiotics as well as other good bacteria in the digestive system.

Most Natural Practitioners would now agree that maintaining good levels of bacteria in your Colon is important for its long term health. Sufferers of Ulcerative Colitis for example are lacking in bifidobacterium, a probiotic strain which is found in large quantities in the bowels of healthy individuals.

In fact if you are suffering from any bowel problem and in particular Inflammatory Bowel Disease, then I recommend to you a new book on probiotics which I have just read. It is written by Peter Cartwright and called 'Probiotics for Crohn's and Colitis' It's available from www.amazon.co.uk

This book goes into detail about the history of probiotics and to a lesser extent, prebiotics. It tells you most of what you need to know about healthy bacteria and its role in the functioning of your bowels.

You can recommend it to your doctor if he is not yet convinced about probiotic supplementation.

Probiotics may be general news now but back in the mid 90's only a few food scientists knew about their importance. They weren't on the radar as far as I was concerned but, once again, because I had been involved in the health trade, I was able to get some good advice and the very first supplement I took was a probiotic formula from the United States.

Unfortunately I found very little benefit even after taking the supplement for more than four weeks. It was clear that my digestive system was running too fast and I guessed that the probiotics I was taking were being flushed straight through as if on a helter skelter.

It was then that I started to look at ways in which I might use soluble fibres to slow down my digestive transit time. Once I started to work with whole psyllium husks I could see some quite instantaneous results. My stools were starting to show proper form and things were getting back to normal.

I did stop taking the probiotics for a while as I wasn't sure if all the benefit was coming from the fibre or a combination of the two ingredients. I soon found out that the whole process worked much better with the inclusion of the probiotics and so I kept taking the two together.

At the time, the probiotics I was taking had to be refrigerated as there was no process for protecting them at normal temperatures, and so it was not possible to carry them around with me whilst travelling.

It was then that I heard about prebiotics. It was this third ingredient that formed the final triangle of ingredients that was going to finally get me back to feeling normal again…

Prebiotics – why not make your own good bacteria?

There are certain extracts of vegetables that act as a fermentable source of food which helps to promote the growth of healthy probiotic bacteria. These extracts are known as inulin and oligofructose.

Inulin is the most studied of prebiotics in recent years. They travel through the digestive system intact and once they enter the large intestine they are converted into friendly bacteria where they start doing their work.

These extracts were eventually given the name of 'Prebiotics' by Professor Gibson at Reading University where much of the recent research has been carried out. One of the advantages that prebiotics have over friendly bacteria is that they are more stable and can survive for longer.

They can also act as a source of food for the friendly bacteria that already exists in your bowels, thus extending their life and activity.

As I have said earlier, onions, leeks, artichokes, and chicory are good sources of prebiotics. However, the level of prebiotics in foods generally is quite small, so taking a prebiotic powder, which is naturally extracted from vegetables, is a good way of helping your system produce more healthy bacteria.

Our ancestors and prebiotics

Our plain-dwelling ancestors were big-time eaters of inulin containing plants and prebiotic consumption was significantly higher than today. The type of subsurface plants and bulbs they used to eat in large quantities were onions and agave. Studies have shown that inulin-rich plants dominated the dietary intake of our ancestors with about 60% of their calorific intake coming from such sources.

This would equal a dietary fibre intake of between 250-400grams and inulin between 50 and 100grams. Today's recommendation is that we should consume between 8 and 10 grams of inulin.

Once again, because of my contacts in the health business, I was able to learn about this wonderful research very early on. It meant that I could take this prebiotic with me on overseas trips as a replacement of the probiotics to enhance the effectiveness of the Psyllium Fibre. The prebiotic powder was totally stable and could be carried in my brief case and this gave me total flexibiltiy.

I found that the combination of fibre and prebiotics worked nearly as well as the probiotic mix and fibre.
However, it wasn't until I mixed the prebiotics and probiotics together, along with the fibre, that I really felt that I had made a total breakthrough.

Ironically, some 10 years later, there is much research underway as to the 'synergistic' benefits of using pro and prebiotics together. It is known as the 'Synbiotic effect' by food scientists.

I do believe that putting these two ingredients together with the fibre is a way of providing the bowels with the best possible food for good health.

How much bacteria do we need overall? This really depends on your levels of health and stress, but for general good health it is recommended that individuals take one billion bacteria daily. This is particularly important for people over 60 as it has been found that beneficial bacteria levels may be reduced a thousand-fold in the elderly. (Curr Opin Clin Nutr Metab Care, 2003: 6: 49-54).

Also, as there are many different types of probiotic bacteria each with a different function, it is recommended that you choose a supplement that contains a number of strains.

So far, I have highlighted three ingredients which can form the basis of a long term health programme for the bowels. In the next session, I am listing four other nutrients which, according to recent studies, may also have benefits for bowel health...

Other nutrients that may benefit your bowel health

There are a growing number of long terms studies going on around the world (which I touched on earlier) looking at our diets and how they can influence our health. I am listing below four nutrients which are emerging as having specific benefit for the health of the bowels and the integrity of the bowel walls.

The bowel wall forms a barrier between the bowels and internal organs, and maintaining its barrier capabilities is vital to preventing it from becoming 'leaky.'

L-glutamine – Your Gut's Best Friend
This is the main fuel required by the intestines for maintenance and repair. Glutamine is an amino acid which reinforces the immune system and there is considerable evidence that it plays a major role in enhancing the barrier function of the gut wall against pathogenic invaders.

Not only does glutamine power your gut, it heals it as well. The cells that make up the inner lining of your digestive tract replace themselves every four days and are your most critical line of defence against developing food allergies or getting infections.

Most health shops have this product in stock in powder form.

Omega 3 Fatty Acids
Omega 3 fatty acids are polyunsaturated fatty acids which the body cannot provide itself. They are known as the 'good fats.' The best known sources are fish oils and flaxseed oil.

Three recent studies, from the UK, Japan and the US have confirmed the protective effect of Omega 3 oils on the bowels, particularly those that are 'sensitive.'

The theory behind this protection is that the fat from fish contains omega 3 fatty acids which are important components of cell membranes. They appear to have anti inflammatory effects and as such have a soothing, gentle action on the intestinal tract.

Good sources of omega 3 are salmon, mackerel, haddock and cod. Flax oil is also a good source.

Calcium

After protein, fat and carbohydrate, calcium in the body has the highest requirement of any nutrient. Milk has often been advocated as the main way of supplying calcium. However, for various reasons, milk is not an option for more and more people.

Several studies have shown that when the levels of Calcium are low, the incidence of bowel disease increases. One study said in order to have a protective effect, you needed to be consuming around 1200mg per day.

Folic Acid

Cells in the digestive tract require folic acid to replicate and heal. One long term study carried out at Harvard Medical School indicated the protective effect of Folic acid against bowel disease.

Folic acid is particularly important for inflammatory bowel problems. The recommended dosage is 40-60mg.

Folic acid is so useful because many people are deficient. It has long been ignored by health authorities and it has only been in recent years that pregnant women have been advised to take it.

Bowel disorders can quite often make it difficult to absorb folic acid so extra is always useful.

Dietary sources are liver, kidney, broccoli, beef, turnips, greens although cooking can destroy it by up to 90%.

So, we've now looked at seven nutrients that can help the health of the bowels. I would now like to offer some tips on two different bowel complaints, sensitive and sluggish bowels...

Some general tips
on sensitive bowels

If your bowels are sensitive and you have not been diagnosed by a doctor for your bowel problem and you are concerned about your symptoms, then it is vital that you make an appointment for an assessment.

Sensitive Bowels can of course range from something as mild as an allergy to certain foods, to something more serious such as Ulcerative Colitis and even Crohns

As a starting point, as my sensitive Irritable Bowel Syndrome problem would fall into this category, I would recommend the combination of whole Psyllium husks, prebiotics and friendly bacteria as the basis for your dietary programme.

The first thing to remember is that the soluble fibre provides bulk and stability to your stools, offering a stable and fertile environment within your bowels for the bacteria to thrive.

It does this by way of the soft gel it forms when mixed with water. You will have read this earlier in the report. Without this stability in the bowels, it can sometimes be hard for the friendly bacteria to survive.

To explain in more detail, this can be demonstrated if your digestive system is running too fast.

In this case, the friendly bacteria can pass straight through offering little or no benefit as there is not sufficient time for it to get established and proliferate. The different strains of bacteria need to have time to establish themselves onto the colon wall.

This is where the fibre comes in. Because of its bulking qualities, Psyllium husk can slow down transit time, giving the pre and probiotics time to flourish and find a 'foot hold' within the colon. Once this takes place, improvements in bowel health can be made.

Also, if your bowels are sensitive, other types of fibre from wheat for example, as I have mentioned earlier, can be far too abrasive and therefore make an already sensitive situation worse.

Your choice of fibre can therefore be very important. If your system has been running too fast for a while then it is likely that your levels of good bacteria are low. The combination of whole psyllium huks, prebiotics and probiotics will hopefully do for you what they did for me.

Sometimes things may get a little worse before they get better, as mucus and other matter that may have impacted on the colon wall is removed.

However, as the system is gradually cleared, if the bacteria can get a hold, then the overall health of your colon should improve. You should find a level of fibre that works for you, always remembering to drink the appropriate amount of water. One teaspoon of Psyllium usually requires 250ml of liquid.

Also it is probably worth trying some form of omega 3 capsules. Eating loads of oily fish is not a bad idea and reducing the consumption of red meat, which can be hard to digest, would also be advisable.

As always, keep your diet as healthy as possible. Antioxidants and nutrients from a healthy diet of vegetables and fruit can offer extra benefit to the bowels.

When your bowels are sensitive, some foods will obviously make it worse. It may be worth looking into possible food allergies. The two obvious ones will be wheat and dairy. However, you may wish to investigate this further with your doctor.

Anything that is obviously fibrous like bran fibre and wheat cereals should be immediately removed from your diet as they will, without question, make an already sensitive situation worse.

One nutrient for the future may be Colostrum. It is generally collected from the first four milkings after calf birth. It is rich in protein, immunoglobulins, lactoferrin and other immune components. Some recent research has indicated that this ingredient may offer benefits for Inflammatory Bowel Disease. Most health shops carry some form of supplement. It is worth reading up on.

So from the too fast to the too slow…

Some general tips on constipation

Although this would appear illogical, Whole Psyllium Husks, as I have mentioned earlier, can also help if your digestive system moves at a Snail's pace as well where waste matter may have been hanging around too long.

The extra bulk the fibre offers gives the bowel wall something to work on, thus encouraging the Peristalsis action. Also, the 'gelling' effect of psyllium and water helps to prevent waste matter from drying up in the bowels and getting too hard, a cause of many bowel problems.

I repeat that a 'moist' stool is far easier and more comfortable to pass. Also, this moist environment that is created by the fibre and water, promotes the type of fertile conditions in which healthy bacteria can flourish, helping to prevent dysbiosis, a situation where bad bacteria gets the upper hand.

The first question you might ask is how often should I go? If you talk to most doctors they would probably say once per day. If you then read an alternative practitioner magazine they will probably say 2 – 3 times per day.

The reality is to try and find some rhythm. Going every two days routinely, provided your stools are well formed, might be ok for some people. However, going daily at least once appears to be the desired target recommended by most specialists.

Finding rhythm might be finding the right time of day to go! Many people feel that mornings are the right time. Clearly if this works for you, then that's great. However, if like many you find mornings can be too rushed to find time and relax, then you might find other times of the day more suitable.

In this case, try making your loo time in the evening when you can relax and take your time. It might take some time to retrain your bowels and find a rhythm but be patient.

I am of course assuming that you are already eating lots of fruit and vegetables and are working towards a Mediterranean diet, but still not having much luck. I do get a lot of people phoning who say that they eat a fresh high fibre diet but their bowels are still very sluggish

I also find that many people I talk to prefer to follow a daily habit with their diets. For example this might mean that they have the same thing for breakfast every day.

My recommendation is to give your body some variety by working out your eating habits over a week, rather than on a daily basis.

So, if you want to improve your bowel transit time, my first recommendation is that you make a list of high fibre foods and try and use these over different days so that you might be taking different types of high fibre foods two or three times per week rather than daily.

Below, I am listing some things that you can 'supplement' your diet with.

- Linseed fibre – this is one of my favourites as it can be added to cereals and mixed in with shakes or smoothies. It is also a good source of essential fatty acids so it is offering other benefits as well.
- Prunes – take 3 times per week.
- Dried fruit such as apricots – take the days you are not taking prunes
- For breakfast have porridge 3 days per week and on other days take other fibre breakfasts, preferably wheat free.
- Vegetables taken raw as 'snacks' are a great way of getting things moving. Most people can cope with raw carrots (even my dog likes them) but raw broccoli is also very effective if you can stomach it raw, but leave out the stalks as they will give you awful wind!
- Lentils are a great source of fibre. They are very versatile and can be added to most things including soup
- Water water water.

Most health shop owners can give good advice on what to take for extra fibre. Often they have good ideas that have been passed on by other customers.

Two other things worth a try are Magnesium Citrate and Digestive Enzymes.

Low levels of Magnesium are often associated with constipation so a month's course of Magnesium Citrate might be worth a try.

Also, if you are over 50, the extra activity of the Digestive Enzymes might be the extra trigger you need to revitalize the digestive system.

Children and constipation

As I mentioned earlier, some hospitals now have constipation clinics for children. I know that many mothers struggle when this situation arises as getting a child to eat healthily can be a problem.

In situations like this, fibre supplementation can help and this is certainly preferable to laxatives.

Psyllium can be too bulky for some children and therefore difficult to take. Instead there are other fibres that might be more suitable. Oats in general are an excellent source of fibre for children. You can now get Oat Beta Glucan in powder form which is an oat fibre that is extracted from whole oats. It can be easily mixed in with soups, shakes and smoothies. Probiotics and Prebiotics should also be considered as they are safe for children to take.

The less fuss you make about their constipation the less stressed your child will be and the better results you will get.

Laxatives

As a general comment, laxatives are OK to use occasionally but if they are used on a long term basis they can be habit forming. Quite often I receive a phone call from someone who has just started taking something like Psyllium and they complain that their bowel movements have not improved.

Further questioning often reveals that this particular person has been on laxatives for a while and have stopped taking them as soon as they start taking the extra fibre. My advice here is to wean yourself off the laxative gradually.

As most laxatives work by stimulation, your system can, over a period of time, get used to them. This means if you suddenly stop taking them the system will close down and stop working for a while until it finds a new rhythm.
How quickly you can rediscover this rhythm will depend on what action you take with your diet.

If you are opting for a new high fibre diet you should stay with the laxative whilst you introduce your new regime.

If you were taking one daily before, then continue to do so. If everything is working fine, then reduce the intake of the laxative to two days. As soon as things are working fine, then go to three days etc. You then need to follow this process until, hopefully, you are off your laxatives completely.